SEXERCISE

OVER
100
TRULY
EXPLOSIVE
TIPS

THIS IS A CARLTON BOOK

Text, illustrations and design copyright © 2002
Carlton Books Limited

This edition published by
Carlton Books Limited 2002
20 Mortimer Street
London W1T 3JW

This book is sold subject to the condition that it shall not, by way of
trade or otherwise, be lent, resold, hired out or otherwise circulated
without the publisher's prior written consent in any form of cover
or binding other than that in which it is published and without
a similar condition including this condition being imposed upon
the subsequent purchaser.

All rights reserved
A CIP catalogue record for this book is available from the British Library
ISBN 1 84222 471 9

Printed and bound in Singapore

Art Director: Penny Stock
Executive Editor: Zia Mattocks
Design: DW Design
Editor: Sian Parkhouse
Production Controller: Janette Davis
Illustrator: Nicola Slater

Neither the author nor the publisher can accept responsibility for
any accident, injury or damage that results from using the ideas,
information or advice offered in this book

SEXERCISE
OVER 100 TRULY EXPLOSIVE TIPS

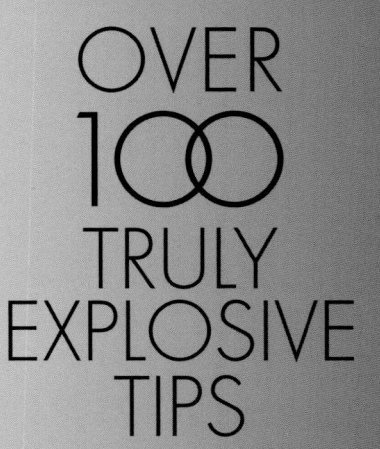

LISA SUSSMAN

CARLTON BOOKS

Section One

WEEK ONE: RECIPES FOR LUST

Your brain may be your most important sexual organ, but there's no getting around the fact that lovemaking gets better when the rest of your body is in shape. Studies on the relationship between sensational sex and health keep coming up with the same finding: just like keeping your car in tip-top condition, the key to a really good sex life (i.e., one that includes not just regular but teeth-rattling orgasms) is proper maintenance.

This isn't about transforming yourself into the female Schwarzenegger; it's about discovering and toning little-known muscles and hormones that contribute to more intense, enjoyable, even transcendent lovemaking for both of you.

The best news is, all it takes to improve your sex life forever is five short weeks. Think you have what it takes to enter the winner's circle? Then look no further for a get-fit plan that will keep you coming – and coming back for more.

Let the games begin!

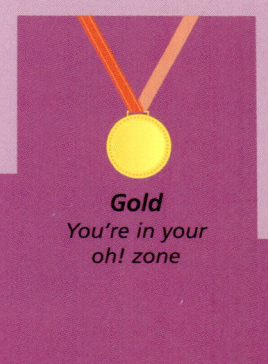

Gold
You're in your oh! zone

Silver
Feel the burn

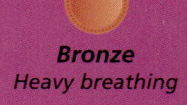

Bronze
Heavy breathing

HORMONE HEAVEN

Getting a grip on your menstrual cycle will help you get the most out of it as a love machine.

Rejoice when your period comes – and not just because it means you're not pregnant. Science has found that those monthly changes in your levels of oestrogen and its sister hormones are what affect the intensity of your orgasms and give you a strong, flexible vagina, and regular production of cervical and vaginal lubricants.

Another happy by-product of following your hormonal peaks is that **oestrogen** and **progesterone** are defenders against STDs within your reproductive tract (although no one's suggesting this means you should skimp on the protection).

Come autumn, **be ready for a quickie**. Hormone levels often peak in October, before they drop again at the first cold spell.

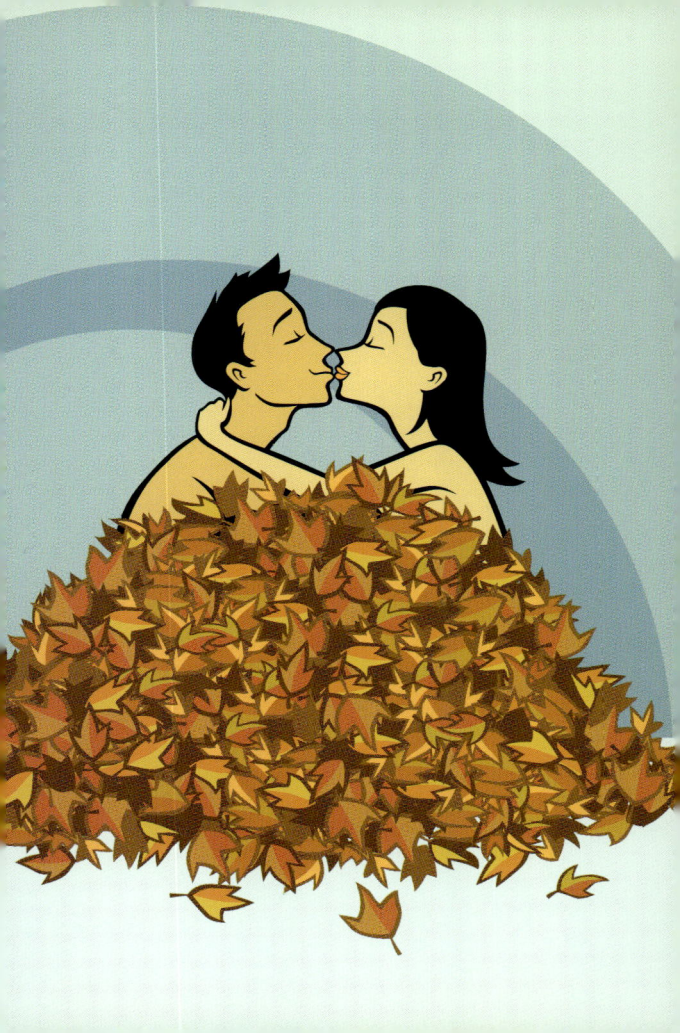

Mark these key days on your calendar:

The average length of a cycle is 28 days. Start counting from the first day of your period.

- It's day 10 and you feel marvellous, darling. Your oestrogen levels are at their pre-ovulatory peak and you are in the mood for love.

- Know where your man is on day 14. It's ovulation time which means testosterone (always present in your blood at a low level) spikes just as oestrogen crests, making you feel sexually aggressive. Your libido's raging and you're at your most man-magnetic. By the way, your body's also primed to get pregnant right now, so don't forget contraception!

- Day 18 and you're in seductive mode – rising levels of oxytocin, the touch hormone, triggers a lust to touch and be touched. Now! Bonus: this hormone also sets off the uterine contractions that go with orgasm.

- Make love on the 28th day of your cycle. Your brain misreads uterine puffiness as a sign of sexual arousal and actually craves orgasmic release. Wowza, wowza!

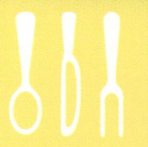

THE PHWOARGASM DIET

This no-deprivation diet will raise your ahhh-q.

5

Honey pollen stimulates reproductive systems. **Swallow the pollen** in tablet form or stir granules straight into food (use those listed in tips 6–9 for a double love whammy).

6

Phosphorus has direct impact on sexual desire. Try food enriched with the miracle mineral (almonds, scallops, cheddar cheese, wheat bran, brewer's yeast and sunflower seeds) for glow-in-the-dark pleasure.

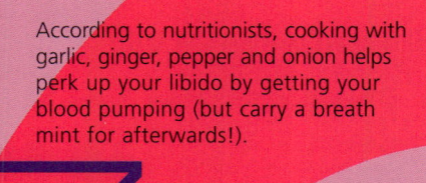

7 According to nutritionists, cooking with garlic, ginger, pepper and onion helps perk up your libido by getting your blood pumping (but carry a breath mint for afterwards!).

8 Vegetarians might just be on to something. Researchers at the US Department of Agriculture have found that the mineral **boron** is vital for hormone production and sexual function. Boron can be found in dark green leafy vegetables, fruits (not citrus), nuts and legumes.

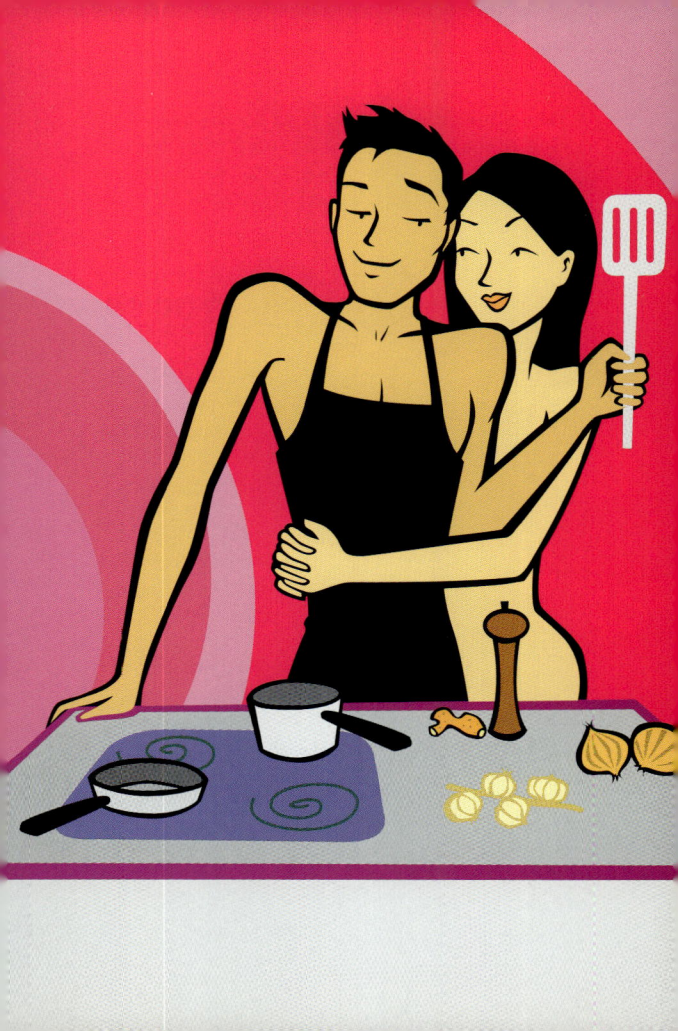

Take your vitamins. You need 45-plus nutrients daily to maintain good health (translation: regular orgasms). Even minor deficiencies can weaken the libido. Here's what you need to stockpile for better bliss. Bon O's.

- Vitamin B (bread, yogurt): converts sugar and starches into energy, which translates into more stamina in bed.

- Vitamin E (spinach, oatmeal, asparagus, eggs, nuts, brown rice, fruit): also known as the sex vitamin, this is the one to pop to perk up passion.

- Zinc (fish, oysters, liver, mushroom, grains, fresh fruit): increases testosterone levels in men and women. University of Rochester researchers found that men with zinc-deficient diets are at high risk for low libido and sex problems like infertility and prostrate problems (his pleasure-zone gland).

- Vitamin D and calcium (milk, cheese): keep bones strong to do tricky positions without embarrassing fractures.

10

Go for a java jolt: a University of Michigan study found that compared to those who did not drink coffee, regular black oil drinkers were considerably more sexually active. Warning: caffeine can also deliver a performance-boosting jolt to sperm cells, increasing both their velocity (speed) and motility (liveliness).

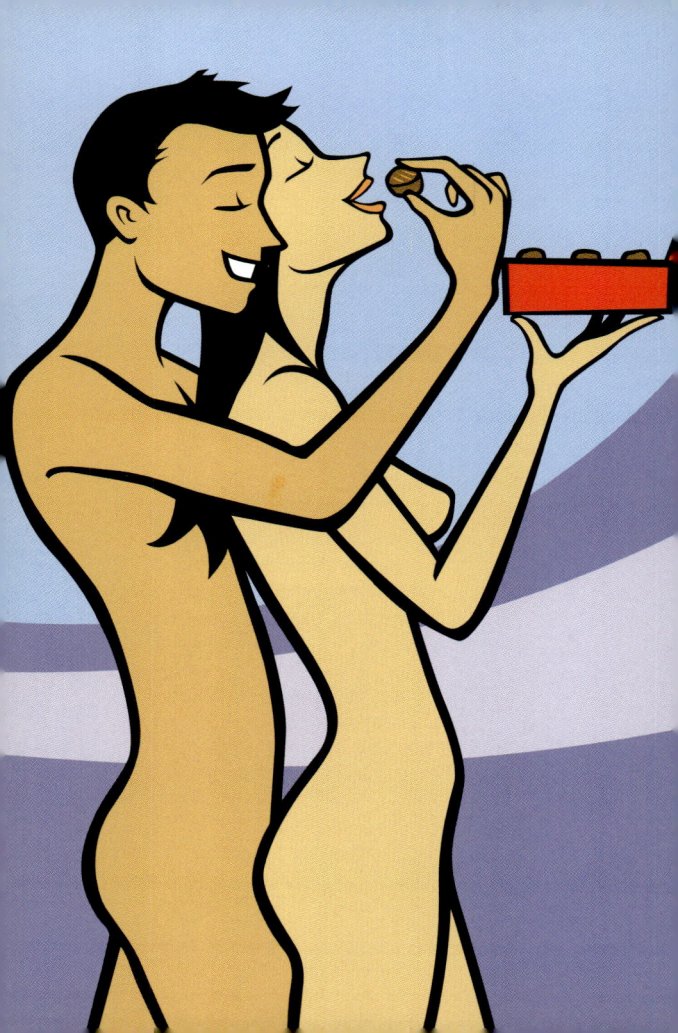

11

Go ahead and eat that Cadbury's. Chocolate contains not only caffeine (see tip 10) but also phenylethylamine (PEA), dubbed the 'molecule of love' by sexual medicine specialist Theresa Crenshaw, MD, author of *The Alchemy of Love and Lust*. A natural form of the stimulant amphetamine, a dose of PEA can increase lust levels to red-hot (the artificial sweetener aspartame also contains PEA so for those watching their weight, a Diet Coke will have the same effect).

LOVE SABOTEURS

Not in the mood? Before blaming your partner, check out your medicine cabinet, diet, birth control and lifestyle.

12

Problem: Fatigue.

Solution: Use your bed … to sleep in, that is. Lots of sex feels great but research shows that you need a minimum of 6–8 hours sleep a night to feel energized for all that sex.

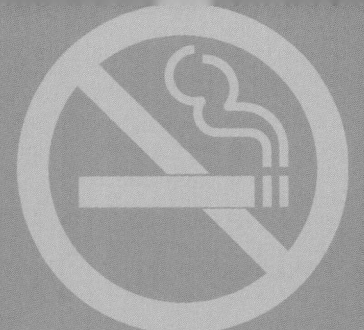

Problem: Smoking.

Solution: Kick ash. It seems that quitting the butt habit can make a bigger difference in your life than exercising. A study at the University of California at San Diego found that tobacco reduces testosterone levels and constricts blood flow, which has a less than smoking effect on your orgasms.

Problem: Contraception.

Solution: Take your pill. A study at McGill University, Montreal, found that Pill users report more frequent and more satisfactory sex than non-users. Possible reasons: lighter menstrual periods, reduced PMS, mental security against pregnancy and the spontaneity of this contraceptive method allows them to relax and enjoy the moment more. (Note: the Pill isn't for everyone – see tip 15 – and should only be used WITH a condom if you aren't sure about your partner's bill of health.)

Problem: The Pill. It contains progesterone, a hormone that diminishes lubrication, sex drive and delays climax. You may still want sex and even enjoy it but the ultimate orgasmic blast-off can become a huge, labour-intensive effort. Hormonal implants can have the same effect.

Solution: Switch to triphasic pills which have different levels of progesterone and, a San Francisco State University study found, may actually even increase desire.

Problem: Your medicine prescription. Research by the Sex/Drug Interaction Foundation in California estimates that up to 20 per cent of all sex problems are caused by drug side effects or interactions. Certain asthma, blood-pressure, diabetes and migraine medications, synthetic androgens (used to treat endometriosis), heartburn soothers, antibiotics and beta blockers (used to treat cardiovascular disease) will all short-circuit desire and orgasm.

Solution: Talk to your doctor about gentler alternative treatments.

Problem: Over-the-counter sex stoppers. Antihistamines, decongestants and sleep aids are muscles relaxants – and you need muscle tension to reach orgasm. In addition, they can dry out the body's mucous membranes, making intercourse uncomfortable.

Solution: Read the label before you buy. If it says, 'May cause drowsiness', it can also impair sexual desire or performance.

Problem: Depression. Selective serotonin re-uptake inhibitors (SSRIs) – like Prozac, Zoloft and Paxil – have been found to have a downing affect on your sexuality, causing lowered libido, lack of arousal, delay in orgasm or reduction in orgasmic intensity.

Solution: A lower dose might reduce sexual side effects while preserving antidepressant effects. Or try a drug holiday (check with your doctor first). A study by MacLean Hospital in Massachusetts found that more than half of those taking antidepressants reported better sexual functioning and more desire when they had drug-free weekends (Thursday noon to Sunday noon). Also see tip 121

19

Problem: Booze. Ironically, we drink to lower inhibition. But alcohol also lowers sex drive. A general rule of thumb is that the amount of alcohol it takes to affect your driving (for an average-size woman, one to two drinks an hour) will also affect your libido.

Solution: Get your high naturally (see tip 121).

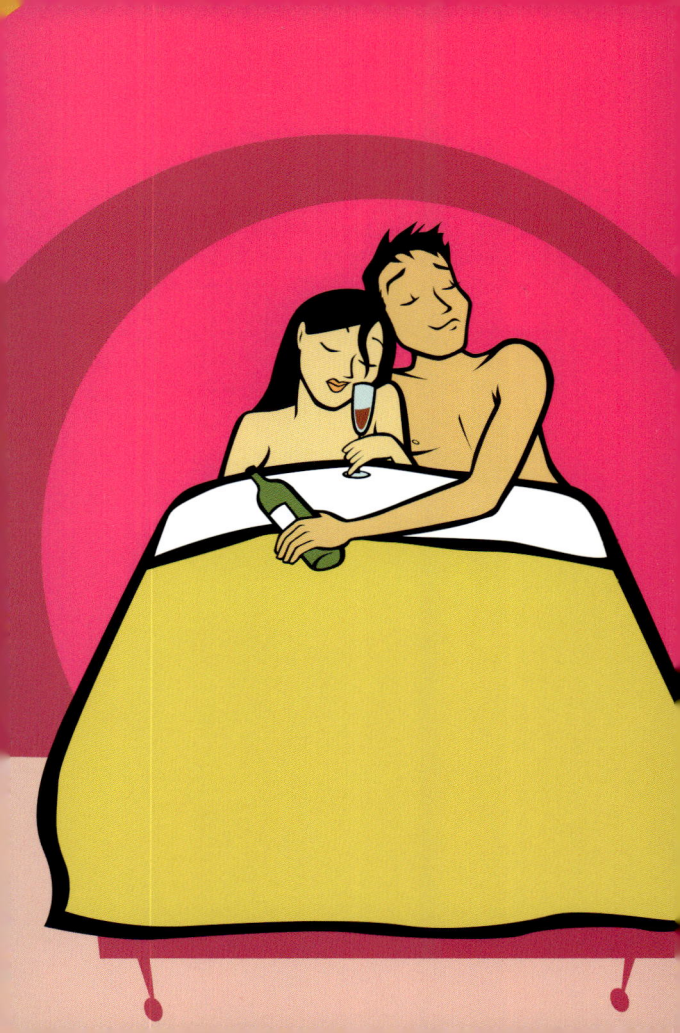

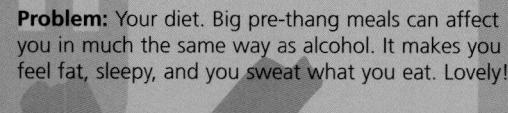

Problem: Your diet. Big pre-thang meals can affect you in much the same way as alcohol. It makes you feel fat, sleepy, and you sweat what you eat. Lovely!

Solution: Lighten up on the heavy meals, especially those containing fatty oils and butter. See tips 5–9 for dishes that'll keep you purring with pleasure.

Problem: His knickers. Besides studies showing that tight briefs might affect his sperm count, lower back moves while wearing tight gym shorts can result in a painful swelling known as stretcher's scrotum.

Solution: Make sure he hangs loose at all times.

Problem: He's a cyclist. Too much wheeling can result in Alcock Syndrome (numb willy from too much bicycle riding).

Solution: Help him get his exercise in other ways (like lying down).

GET NATURAL

Additive free doses of desire.*

Gingko biloba
WHAT IT DOES: Several studies have found that it improves blood flow throughout the body by relaxing arteries, aiding potency in men and orgasmic release in women.
DOSE: Start at 80 mg per day.

Ginseng
WHAT IT DOES: This herb contains ginsenosides, compounds that researchers think can improve sexual function by encouraging the body to make more testosterone.
DOSE: 2 g per day. Be sure to check the label for the designation Panax, which means that the herb is of American or Oriental origin (the most reliable). It's also important to buy a standardized formula containing 15 per cent ginsenosides; that means the manufacturers have tested the product to ensure that there are sufficient quantities of the active ingredient.

*Warning: You may have to take these herbs for several weeks before you see any results. Let your doctor know what you're taking to avoid interactions with other medications and never take any herbs if you are pregnant.

Avena sativa
WHAT IT DOES: This green oat straw has been a staple of sex formulas because it may help alleviate sexual problems (especially low libido) by raising testosterone levels. In one study, 20 men who took the extract reported a 54 per cent increase in frequency of sexual activity.
DOSE: 300 mg per day

St John's wort
WHAT IT DOES: A natural antidepressant, it is also thought to be a natural libido lifter. Warning: It's been found to decrease the effectiveness of the Pill.
DOSE: 900 mg per day of a 0.3 per cent standardized extract.

Damiana
WHAT IT DOES: This herb has a long-standing reputation as a sexual stimulant. It contains volatile oils that stimulate nerve endings and increase circulation to the genitals.
DOSE: Steep two teaspoons of fried damiana leaves in one cup of water and drink three times a day.

Section Two

WEEK TWO: THE LOVE WORKOUT

Ever tried a new position, only to find that while the mind is willing, the thighs are screaming, 'How long do you expect me to keep this up?' Unlike most full-contact sports, you can't call time-out during lovemaking. Which is why trimming the flab, toning muscles and building stamina are vital to getting good sex (good hygiene and ace blow job skills don't hurt either). An orgasm is essentially a series of contractions of the uterine, vaginal, rectal and pubococcygeus (PC) muscles. Ergo, the stronger your muscles, the stronger the contractions, the more pleasure you'll feel and the more control you'll have over your own – and your lover's – bliss.

All it takes is 20 minutes of exercise a week to develop killer love muscles. Keep it moderate (around 145 heartbeats per minute) or you'll be too whacked to get whacked. Expect results within weeks.

One word of caution all you A-type personalities: take it easy. In the sex/exercise connection, more isn't better (good news). Too much muscles soreness and fatigue can easily put a damper on romance while over-rigorous training can cause hormonal imbalances in your libido. Three times a week is more than enough to feel results.

JUST DO IT

It's official: A hard body leads to better whoa!

It starts with the heart. In a study of nearly 3,000 men and women by the University of California at San Diego, it was found that as fitness levels improve, so does cardiovascular endurance. This means a greater volume of blood can be pumped throughout the body – genitals included. And blood circulation is key for a man's erection and a woman's arousal system (it increases lubrication and clitoral swelling). Kinda makes you want to check out those step classes after all, huh?

29

Don't be afraid to break a sweat – perspiration is actually an aphrodisiac packed with come-hither-and-ravage-me pheromones (up the stakes by chucking away your deodorant). In Shakespeare's time, a woman hoping to attract a man tucked a peeled apple in her armpit and then offered this 'love apple' to the object of her lust.

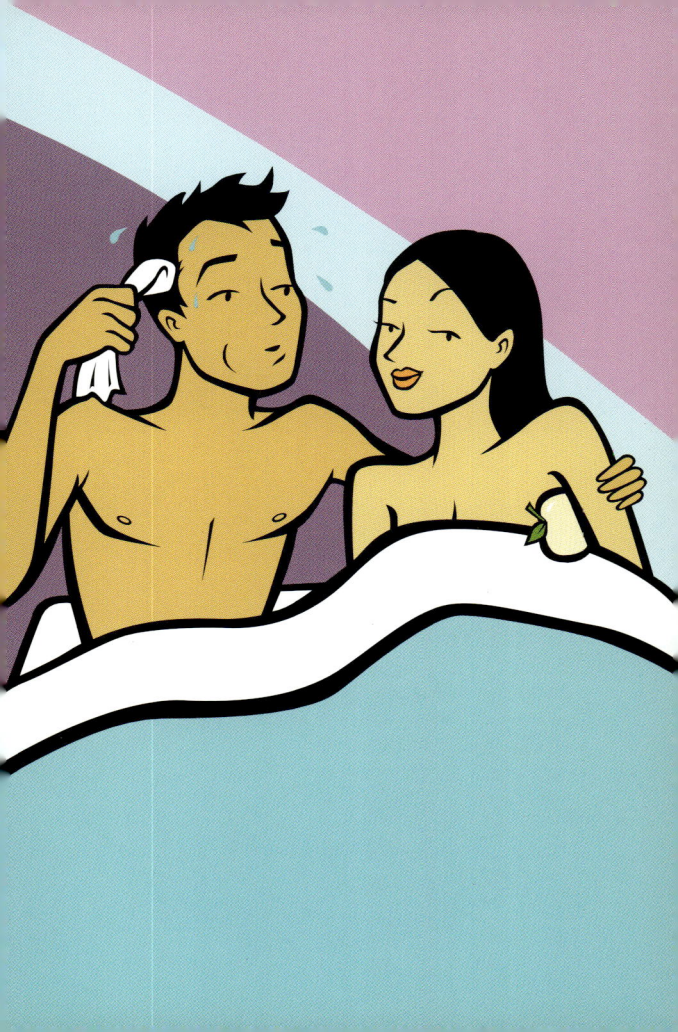

30

Another reason to skip your **post-workout shower** and steam up in bed instead: exercise also stimulates the endocrine glands, making testosterone levels in both men and women rise sharply. Translation: you want it and you want it now.

3

Additional bonus: if you're healthy and in good shape, you may climax more easily. Sex therapist Dr Linda De Villers studied more than 8,000 women and found regular exercisers had more intense and fulfilling orgasms – perhaps because people who workout take pride in their bodies and have higher self-esteem. (It's harder to have an orgasm if you're obsessing over the size of your bum.)

If the above still hasn't made you jump on a treadmill, consider this: pumping it up also gets you in shape for your own tour de sex. Regular aerobic activity – such as cycling, swimming, jogging or stepping on a Stairmaster – improves cardiovascular endurance, which translates to **more staying power in the bedroom**.

And don't forget the **curative powers** of exercise. For years, women who had problems with sex drive, arousal or orgasm were told to relax and take a bubble bath. But research from the University of Texas at Austin suggests the opposite is true: women should do something arousing to get stimulated – like working out. Get revved. Time to renew that gym membership?

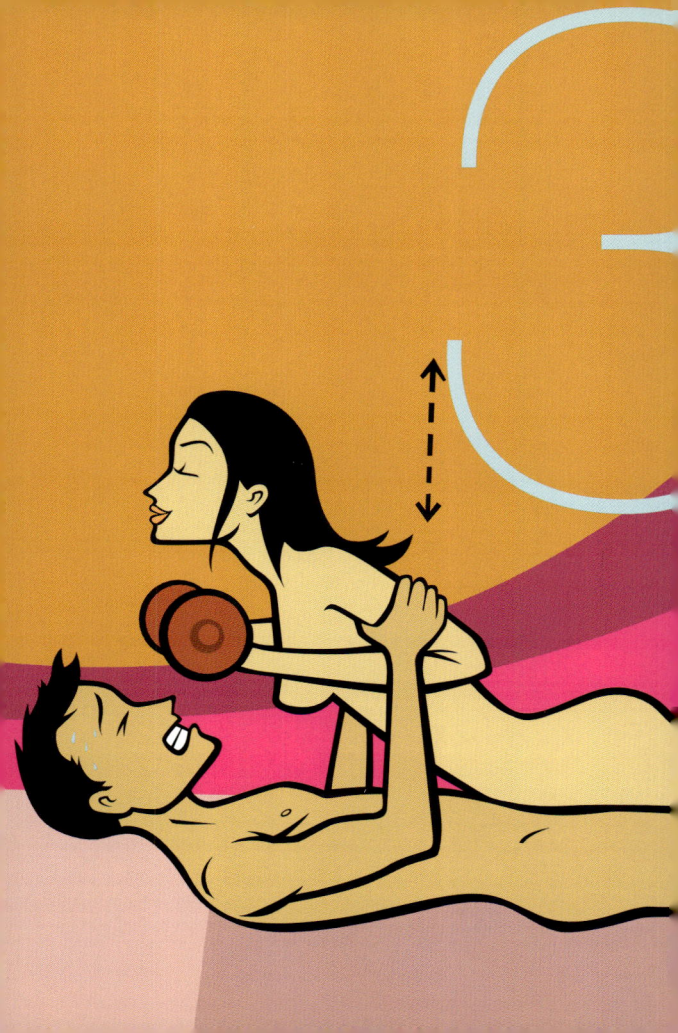

34

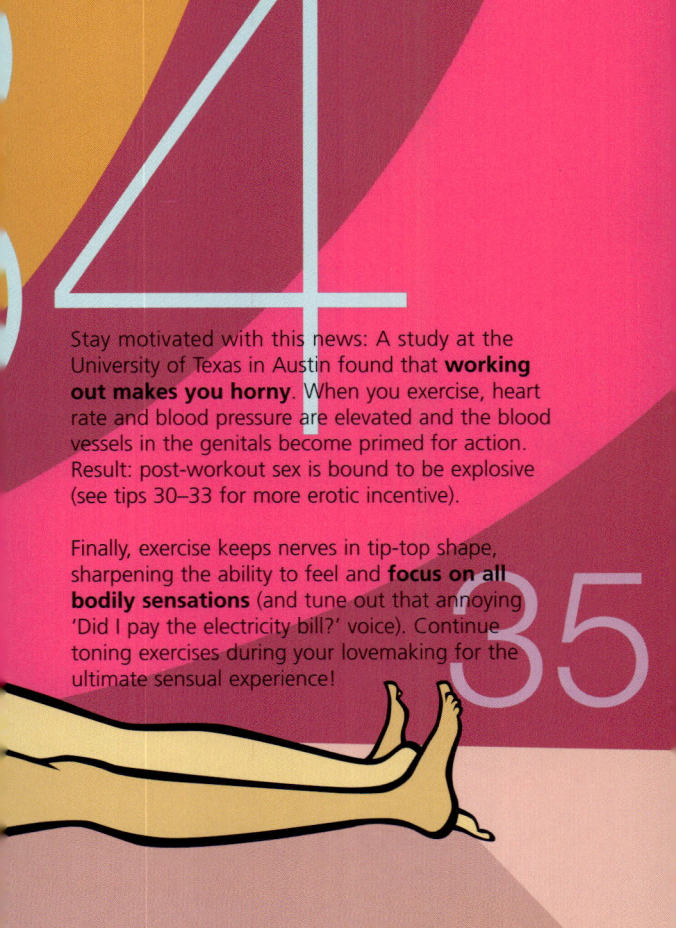

Stay motivated with this news: A study at the University of Texas in Austin found that **working out makes you horny**. When you exercise, heart rate and blood pressure are elevated and the blood vessels in the genitals become primed for action. Result: post-workout sex is bound to be explosive (see tips 30–33 for more erotic incentive).

35

Finally, exercise keeps nerves in tip-top shape, sharpening the ability to feel and **focus on all bodily sensations** (and tune out that annoying 'Did I pay the electricity bill?' voice). Continue toning exercises during your lovemaking for the ultimate sensual experience!

Don't leave him on the couch: after nine months of working out for one hour three times a week, your man is likely to have a shorter post-ejaculation recovery period. Hello, orgasmic hat tricks!

Don't leave him on the couch 2: The American Council on Exercise reports that burning at least 200 calories a day exercising (the equivalent of walking two miles briskly) can keep his willy perky and interested, preventing or even reversing premature ejaculation, low libido and penile droop.

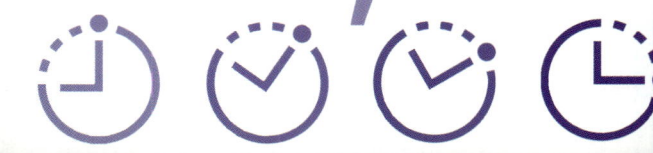

SWEAT IT OUT

Key cardio moves for getting hot and bothered.

Alternate your aerobic days with a weight-training regimen that covers the full body – arms, legs, abdomen, chest and back (see tips 48–51, 55, 56 and 83 for ideas). Use either free weights or a weight machine system like Nautilus. The goal is to **increase strength and tone muscles**, so work with a weight that's about half of what you're capable of lifting. Do three sets of 12 repetitions for each muscle group.

39

Start pounding the pavement. In one poll, 66 per cent of the men and women runners interviewed claimed that regular jogging made them better lovers.

40

Or **put a spin** on your workouts. In another poll, two-thirds of bicycling enthusiasts said cycling made them better lovers.

41

Lap it up for long-lasting juiciness. A Harvard University study of middle-aged swimmers concluded that men and women over 40 who got wet regularly were as sexually active as people in their late twenties and early thirties. And they enjoyed it more.

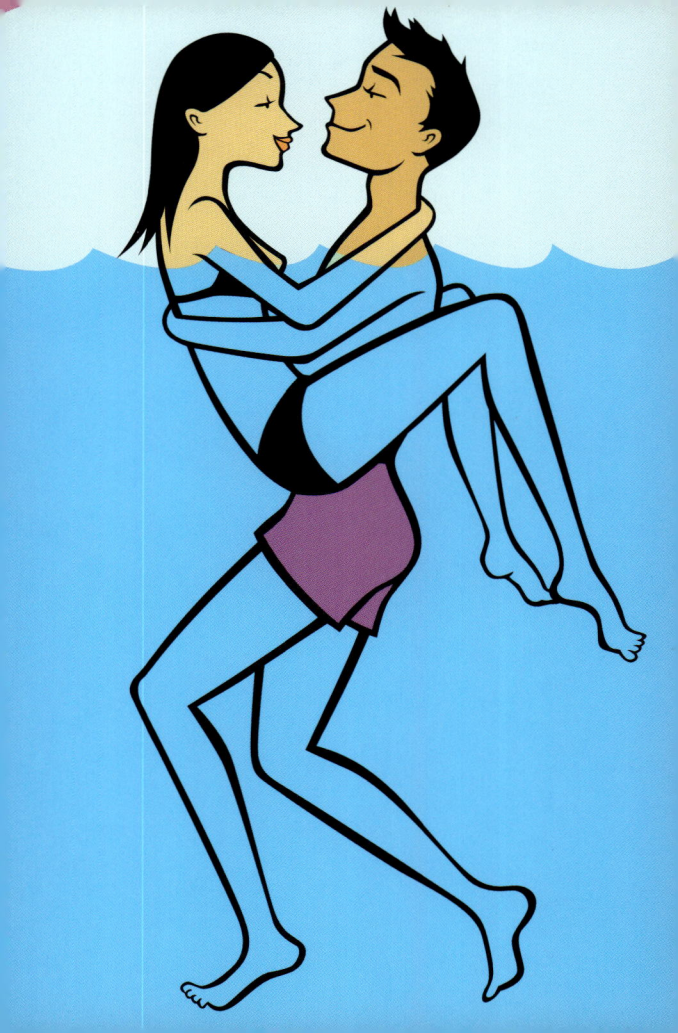

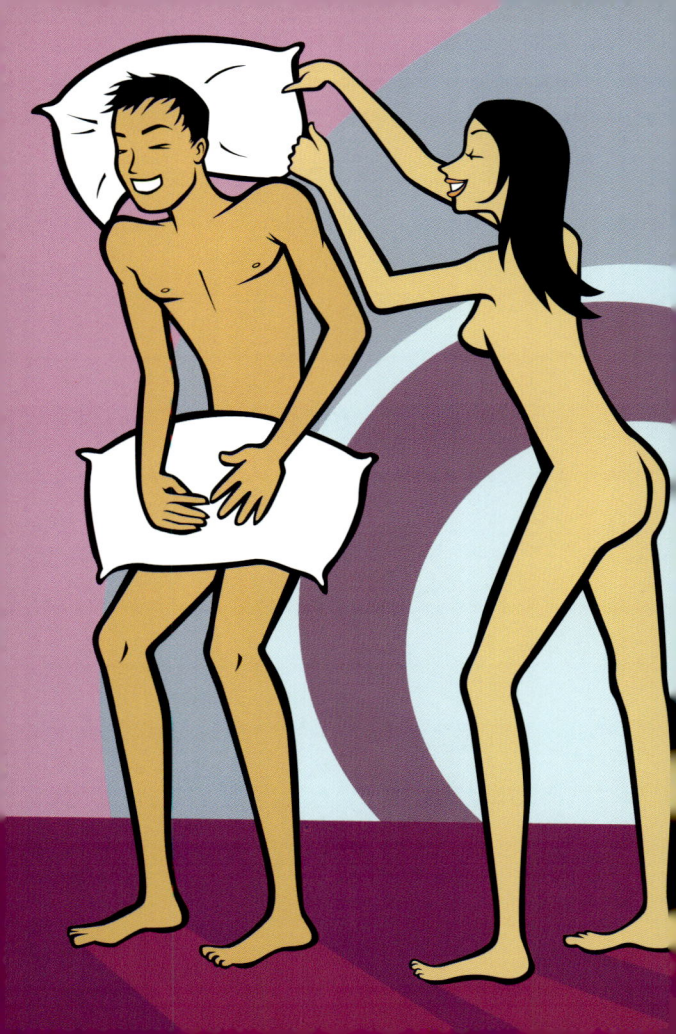

42

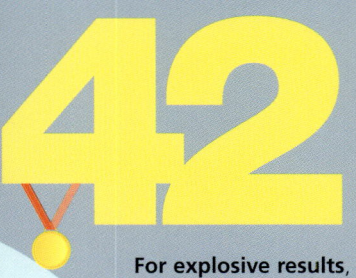

For explosive results, go from almost no exercise to three one-hour workouts a week. One study found that this technique results in a 30 per cent increase in how often you play the field, a 20 per cent increase in tonsil hockey and a decrease in being benched because of non-working parts.

Insider tip: you don't have to schedule a gym trip every time you want to have sex. The kind of breathlessness necessary for a **precoital charge** can also be had from a rowdy, bawdy pillow fight with your lover. Tickling, wrestling and fighting can all also set off sparks.

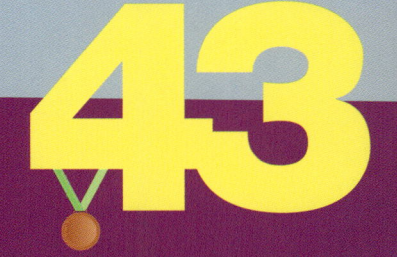

43

PELVIS POWER

Forget upper arms as taut as cables and a bum so firm you can flip a coin off of it – the stronger your and his pelvic muscles are, the tighter you'll both be able to contract during sex and squeeze out every last drop of pleasure (see tips 77–81 for more on how to apply penile pressure).

Libido lifter: Lie flat with your arms at your sides, knees bent and feet flat on the floor. Raise your hips as high as you can and hold for a count of three, then lower them until your body nearly touches the floor. Do triple sets of ten three times a week for pumping endurance that a WWF wrestler would envy.

45

The thrust: A variation of tip 44. Lie down as before, then raise your hips so your bum is the only part of your body off the floor. Slowly rock or tilt your pelvis up while exhaling and down while inhaling. Repeat slowly and smoothly 20 times.

The tilt: Open the muscles of the pelvic floor by getting down on all fours with your hands directly beneath your shoulders and your knees under your hips. On a long, slow inhalation, lower your belly and lift your pelvis, then look towards the ceiling. On the exhalation, arch your back upwards, drop your head and tuck your tailbone forward. Slowly and smoothly alternate between these poses for about 30 seconds, focusing on the movement in your pelvis.

Rock-and-roll: Stand and swivel your hips, doing a rolling motion as if you're doing a bad Elvis imitation. Move only your hips, not your shoulders or upper body. Do this for one or two minutes at various speeds once or twice a day.

LIFT IT

Before you do the limbo of love, beef up with these never-gruelling-always-gratifying strength-training moves that target your erotic core. (Don't worry – they take longer to read than to actually do.)

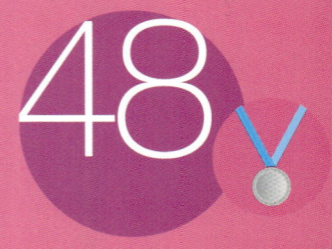

48

Shoulders: To keep you in shape for staying on top (which is, incidentally, the best position to stimulate the G-spot and other sensitive areas in the vagina, such as its end).

WORK IT: Sit up. Hold your arms above your head and cross your wrists. Inhale, straightening your arms. Extend them back behind your head as far as possible, keeping your wrists crossed (your elbows should be behind your ears). Hold for ten seconds, then relax. Repeat three times.

MIX IT IN: See tips 83, 84 and 91.

Upper arms: Strengthening the triceps will help you hold yourself up longer when you're on top (see tip 48 for why you want to be on top).

WORK IT: Sit on a chair with its back against a wall, holding the front of the seat with the heels of your hands. Slide off the chair and freeze, with your knees bent, elbows facing the wall and arms supporting your body. Lower your body, bending your elbows to a 90° angle, then push up. Do 3 sets of 15.

MIX IT IN: See tips 83, 89 and 92.

49

Abdominals: These are your orgasmic power centre. They help maintain your position, push your inner clitoris into the path of his penis, keep the lower back strong (important for those sexy thrusts) and hold your belly in (important when it comes to luring a partner to willingly do the aforementioned thrusting motions with you).

WORK IT: Sit up straight. Pull your belly button in for one second, imagining it's touching back of your spine. Release. Repeat 99 times, counting aloud (so you don't hold your breath). Aim for five sets of 100 a day.

MIX IT IN: Squeeze your abs during sex – you'll beef up your orgasms to twice their usual size (see tips 85 and 88 for more fabdominal ideas).

Derrière: Strengthening these muscles helps build pressure in your pelvic region – which will feel incredible when released.

WORK IT: Flex and release your bum rhythmically for about 20 seconds every day.

MIX IT IN: Clenching your buns together every couple of seconds during sex will push you both over the Big O brink (see tip 95 for more yum-bum moves).

52

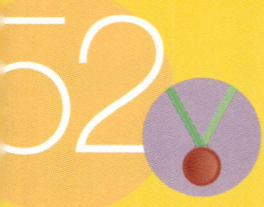

Back: Sex feels better than busting concrete, but your back muscles don't know the difference. Sex-related backaches are especially common when nearing climax, the point of maximum muscle tension.

WORK IT: Lie on your back and slowly bring your knees to your chest. Grab your knees and hold them against your chest for a few breaths, relaxing throughout the movement.

MIX IT IN: Elevate your legs by lying flat on the floor and propping your feet on the backs of his thighs during sex. This will take the pressure off the sciatic nerve and relax those hot twinges of a minor backache. Tips 84 and 88 will also make you sit straight with pleasure.

Hips: Don't forget to hit below the belt. As the key pivot in the thrusting motion, your hip joint and muscles must remain flexible.

WORK IT: Push both thighs outwards and hold for thirty seconds. Relax. Repeat ten times.

MIX IT IN: Get on top – it's an instant hip easer (see tip 83 for muscle workers to stay on top).

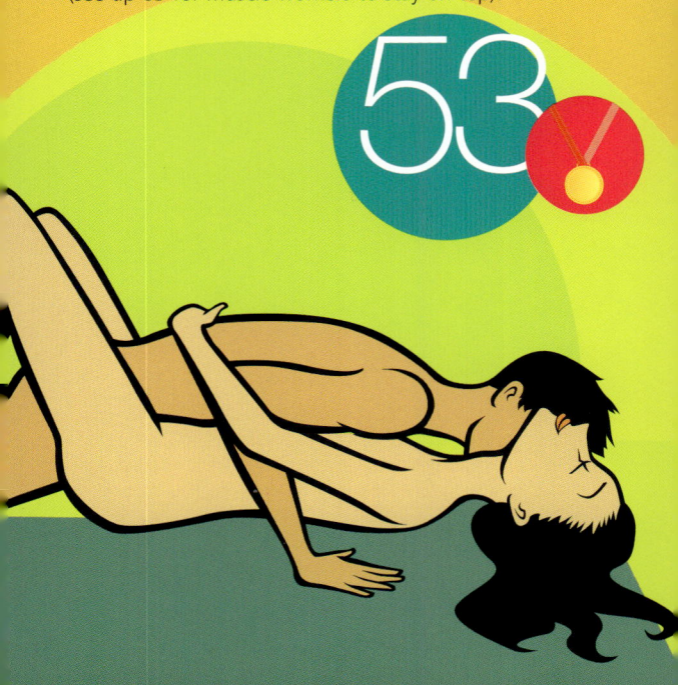

53

54

Inner thighs: Necessary for those tricky standing-on-one-leg-on-a-tree-limb moves.

WORK IT: Sit on a chair and squeeze your knees, pushing them together for about ten seconds. Repeat ten times, three times a day.

MIX IT IN: Do the squeeze during the missionary position – you'll create friction on the outer part of the clitoris and the inner folds of the vulva – yum!

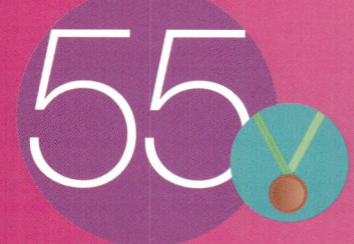

55

Upper thighs: The quads – the muscles at the front of the thighs – are key players in any on-top position (see tip 48 for why you want to train for this position).

WORK IT: Stand 30 cm (1 ft) away from a wall, facing out. Lean back so your torso touches the wall. Slide down, bending your knees until your thighs are parallel to the floor. Hold for 30 seconds, building up to two minutes.

MIX IT IN: Check tip 96 to put these muscles in use.

56

Calves: This move stops you from overflexing your calf muscles during orgasm (and ending up with the wrong kind of spasms).

WORK IT: Lie flat on your back with one leg bent and one leg straight. Raise the straight leg as far as you can until it's pointing at the ceiling. Hold and exhale while slowly flexing your foot, pointing the toes down towards your chest. Relax, then lower the leg. Repeat three times on each leg.

MIX IT IN: Lock your legs around his hips and squeeze your calves, drawing him closer.

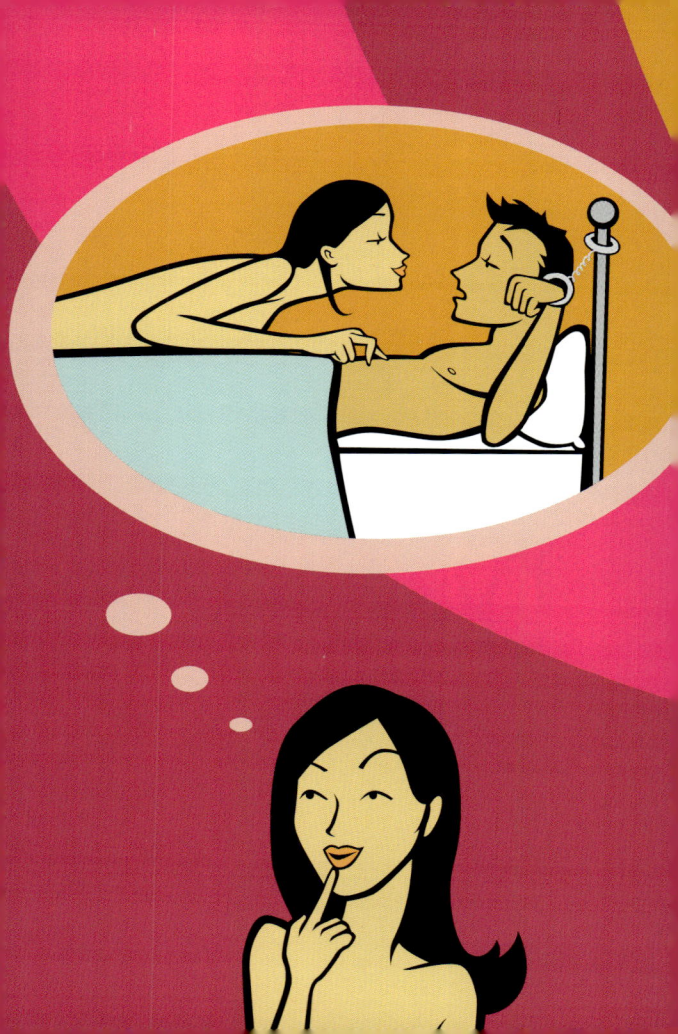

Brain: This is your main love muscle, so go for the golden goal and keep it strong.

WORK IT: Fantasize, dream up new scenarios and ways to touch him.

MIX IT IN: Share the above with your lover.

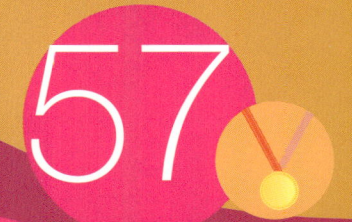

57

Section Three

WEEK THREE: THE JOY OF FLEX

It's not enough to be strong. You also want to be limber and loose. Studies have found that muscle tightness dramatically blocks the range of motion of the legs, hips and pelvis – all key players in sexual activity. In addition, most of us clench our muscles when aroused, trying to almost push ourselves into coming.

On the flip side, stretching pumps a lot of blood into muscles and that stimulates the nerves that run through them. And when you can relax and go slack and submit to ecstasy, your orgasm will simply come to you.

These stretches and breathing exercises will help you loosen up for every tight spot you want to get in. Designed to stretch and tone AND make you both moan, these should be done two or three times weekly to stay permanently loose or within several hours of a planned rendezvous to help you soar to a more aware and prolonged state of arousal.

58 GET A BUZZ ON

Breathe your way to erotic bliss.

To make it through the long haul, long-distance runners must learn to master their breathing. And if you want to make medal-winning moves on your mattress, you should do the same. Breathe deeply through your mouth, all the way down to your diaphragm. Once you have a rhythm going, speed it up breath by breath to raise the level of sexual excitement and push you over the finishing line.

Learn the seven chakra breaths. Inhale deeply so that your lower belly expands. Exhale slowly and fully, using the abdominal muscles to expel all of the air from the lungs. With each complete breath (inhale plus exhale), focus on the base of your spine (strength), uterus (sexuality), stomach (emotions), heart (love), throat (expression), forehead (intuition), and crown (individuality). This will open up all the places where there's tension, enhancing sensitivity, allowing pleasure in, heightening sexual perceptions and increasing stamina. Make love immediately after doing this – it's more likely you'll have a whole body orgasm.

This only works when you know you're **about to get lucky**. Plug your left nostril for fifteen minutes prior to the action starting and you'll increase the air flow to the sexier side of the brain, which really gets you in the mood. Of course, that tissue dangling from your nose might kill it.

Share a Tantric kiss: Sit on his lap. Inhale while he's exhaling. As he breathes out, you'll suck his breath into your body, down to your sex organs. After one minute, kiss and share your breath. Intercourse may not even be necessary when you're so merged.

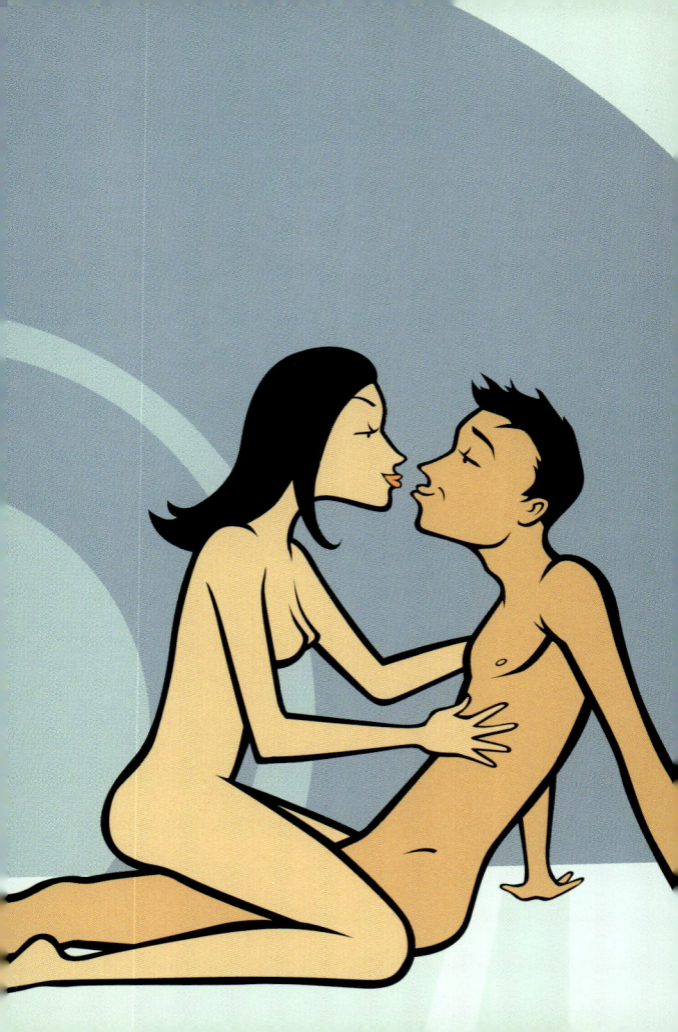

STRETCH YOURSELF SEXY

Prepare for passion with these lusty moves to improve your let-me-at-him lunges.

Imagine the **positions you want** to get in for lovemaking and do them as stretches. Hold the pose, breathing deeply and stretching just a little more with each exhale.

The psoas muscle is central for **rocking the pelvis forward** and back and side to side – moves that turn sex into an ooh-la-la experience. Strengthen yours with this yoga stretch. Stand with your knees slightly bent and inhale while gently rocking your pelvis back. Exhale as you smoothly return to your original position. Your weight should remain evenly balanced on your feet.

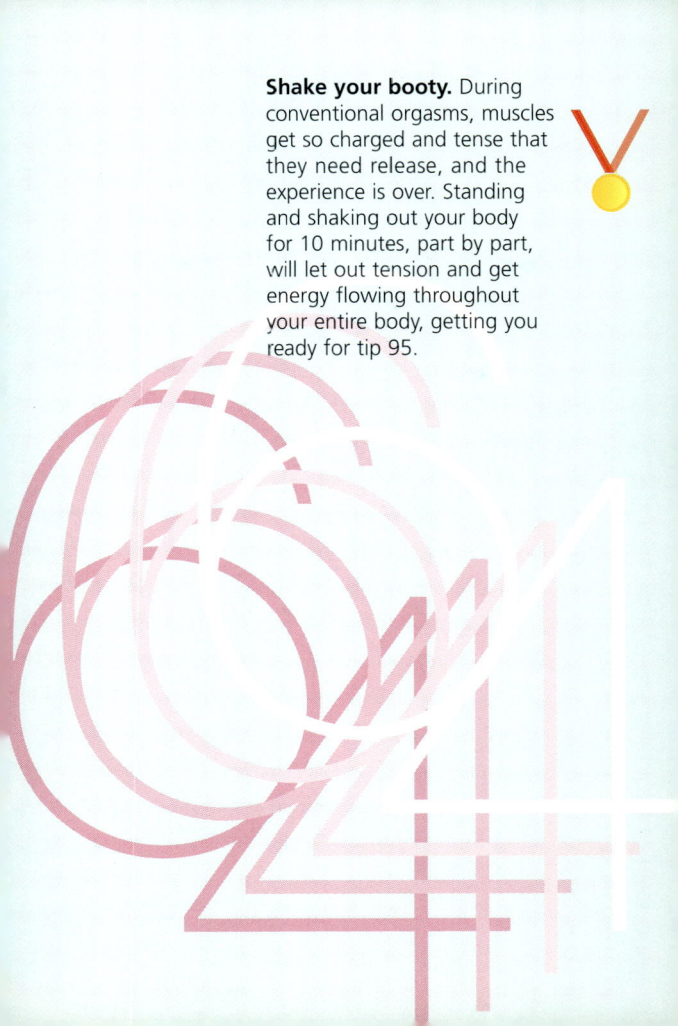

Shake your booty. During conventional orgasms, muscles get so charged and tense that they need release, and the experience is over. Standing and shaking out your body for 10 minutes, part by part, will let out tension and get energy flowing throughout your entire body, getting you ready for tip 95.

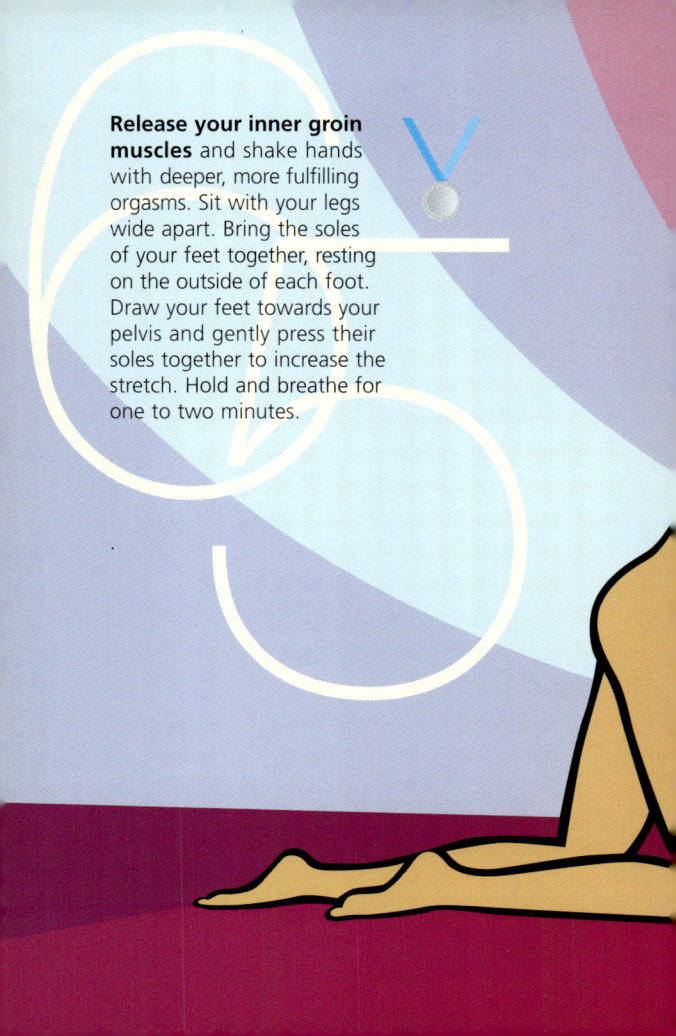

Release your inner groin muscles and shake hands with deeper, more fulfilling orgasms. Sit with your legs wide apart. Bring the soles of your feet together, resting on the outside of each foot. Draw your feet towards your pelvis and gently press their soles together to increase the stretch. Hold and breathe for one to two minutes.

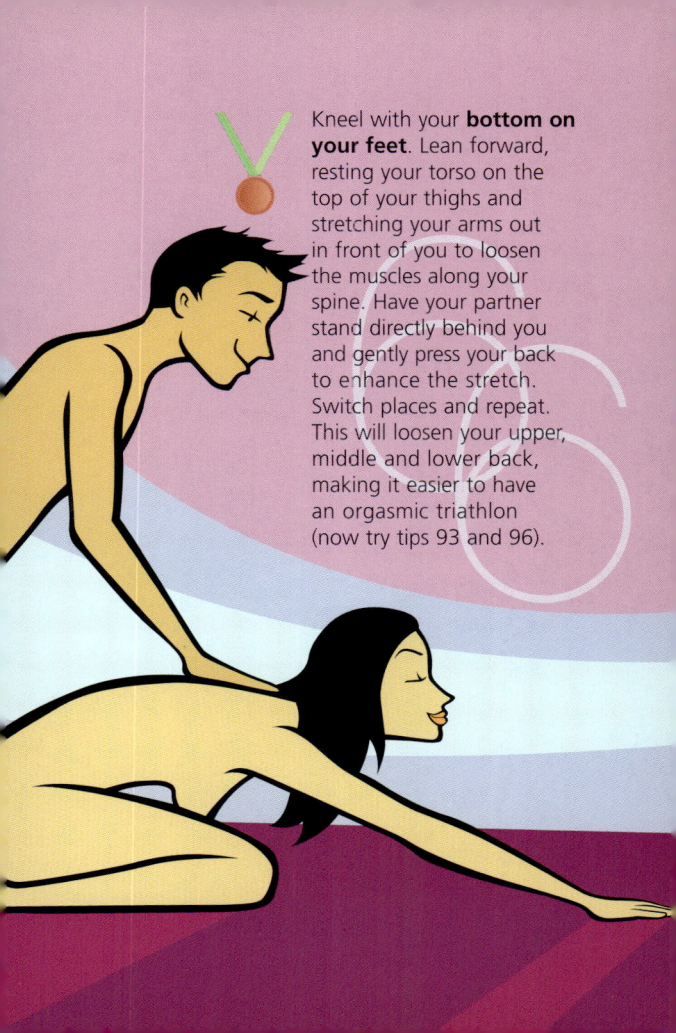

Kneel with your **bottom on your feet**. Lean forward, resting your torso on the top of your thighs and stretching your arms out in front of you to loosen the muscles along your spine. Have your partner stand directly behind you and gently press your back to enhance the stretch. Switch places and repeat. This will loosen your upper, middle and lower back, making it easier to have an orgasmic triathlon (now try tips 93 and 96).

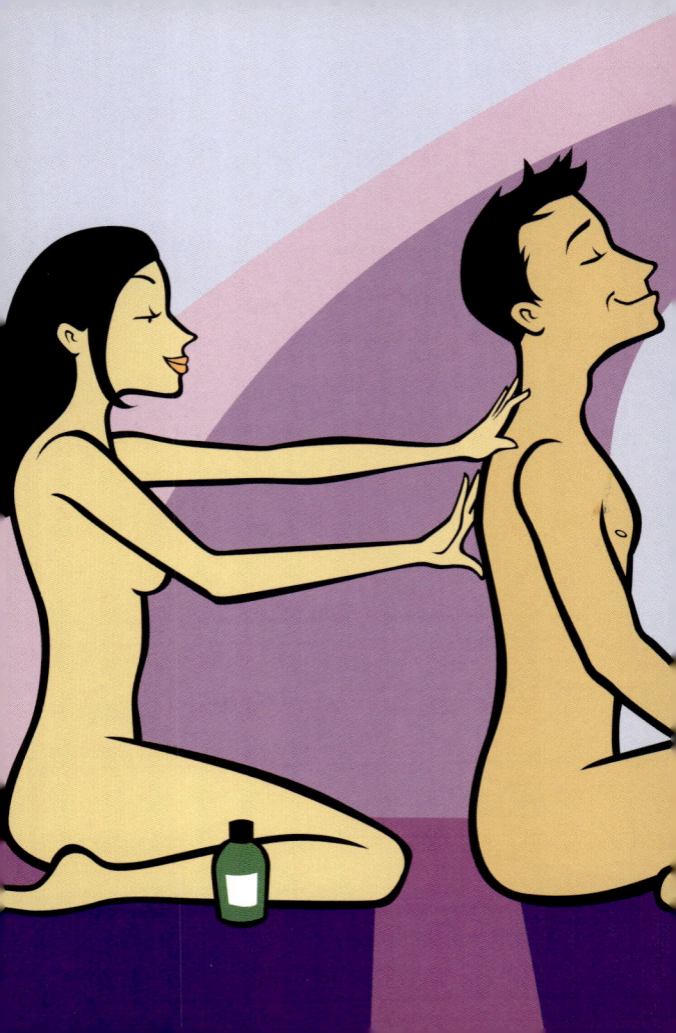

Get a quick lift when you feel drained by lowering your head, flipping your hair forward and pressing on the back of your head. This area is your energy zone and stretching it boosts circulation (the secret to all good orgasms). Extra pick-you-up-and-push-you-over-the-edge tip: spritz the area with a sharp, spicy fragrance containing musk or ylang ylang.

Knead out those knots. A sensual massage will turn up the body heat in more ways than one. Athletes get massages to increase circulation to the muscle groups. The increased blood flow warms the muscles so they'll stretch more easily and perform to their fullest capacity. To ensure personal-best sexual performance, dab a few drops of massage oil or lotion on your hands and place them, palms flat, on your partner's lower back. Run your palms in small circles up his back, along both sides of his spine, all the way up to his shoulders. Have him do the same for you. Then slip yourselves into tip 97.

GET SPIRITUAL

Shape up with this no-sweat Tantric workout. For best results, follow it step-by-step.

Connect: dim the lights, then sit facing each other, gazing into each other's eyes for at least five minutes.

69

70

Lay head-to-head on the floor so that your legs form one long line. Nestle your heads on each other's shoulders. The goal is to relax and tune into each other until you can breathe together – it'll take about ten minutes (see tip 59 for more on heavy breathing).

Sit facing each other and redo tip 69.

71

72

Place your hands on each other's chests, **feeling both your hearts beat**. Breathe (see tip 58 for hot panting).

Kiss. Taste each other everywhere. When you become really excited, though, stop and return to tip 69. It's important not to work up too much of a sweat – Tantric-style sex is calm and restful. The point is to keep your head clear while your body gets completely turned on.

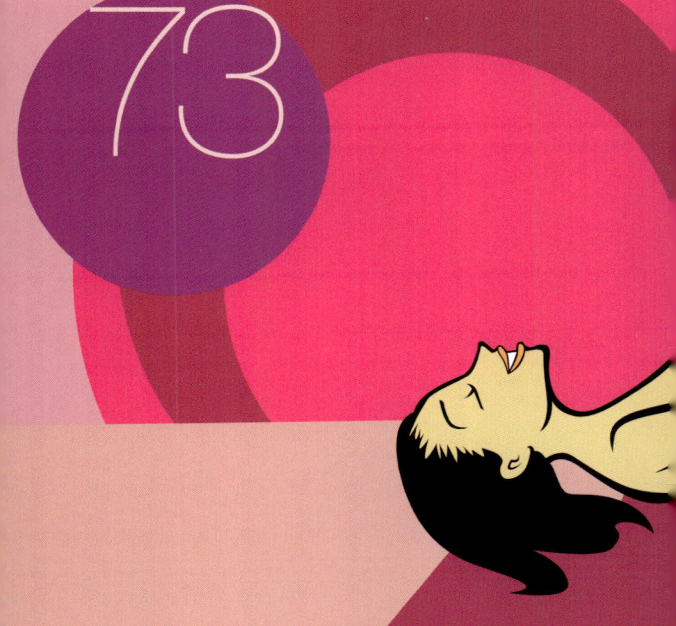

73

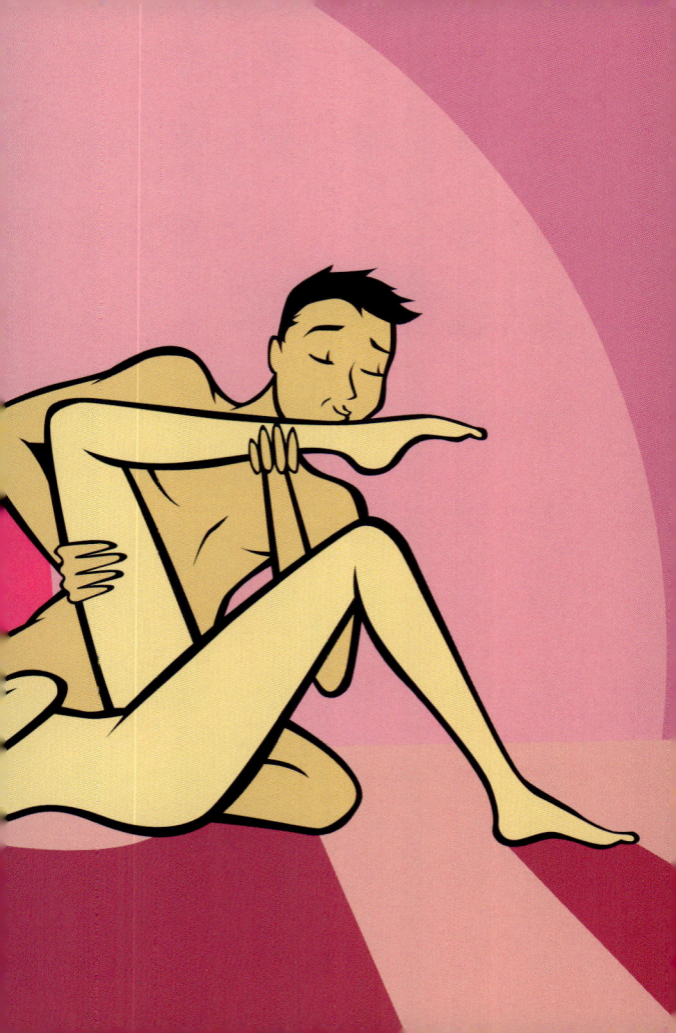

Almost do it, position 1: Get into your O-Zone – get on top with your body resting on his chest and your shins flat on the mattress. He enters you partially – an inch every five minutes (don't measure!). Lay still as long as you can. Do your Kegels (see tip 77) to help him stay erect. When you can't take it any more, start stroking and kissing (see tip 61 to make this even sexier), but stop after 20 minutes, letting your bodies go limp so you don't come.

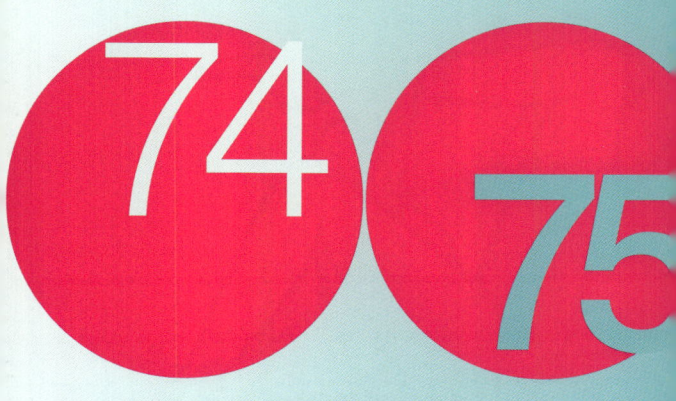

74

75

Almost do it, position 2: He lays on his side (if you're using condoms, this is the time to put on a new one) while you lay on your back with your legs over his and your bodies at a 45° angle. Start again from tip 69. When you get to step 72, go limp again (see tip 73).

Now really do it, position 3: Repeat tips 69–72. Then sit on his lap so that you're facing him. This time, let yourself go completely for a total gut-busting orgasm that will stay with you for days.

76

Section Four

WEEK FOUR: THE INTERCOURSE ORGASM

Time to use the greatest piece of fitness equipment ever invented: a bed.

Anyone who's limber, toned and in shape can make love like a rabbit. But sex is more like synchronized swimming than a 100-metre dash. Timing, in other words, is everything. Bottom line: a strong tongue muscle is only going to get you so far between the sheets. What you need to do is add some exercises and stretches that target the parts of the body called into play during lovemaking, giving you more control over and more intensity during your orgasm. These following high-voltage moves will help boost your performance and give your sex life more pleasure than a lifetime supply of sex toys.

PUMP IT UP

Studies have found that stronger pubococcygeus (PC) muscles make women more orgasmic more frequently and men more likely to experience multiple orgasms. Enough said – here's how to do them.

Squeezing your PCs is a bit like wiggling your ears – if you've never focused on the sensation before, finding these muscles may take a bit of time. Here's your four-step guide to gold-standard love muscles:

- The easiest way to locate your PCs is to try to stop your urine flow while on the loo (don't do this more than once a day, as it may irritate your bladder).
- Once you have a general idea of where your PC is, practise the basic Kegel exercise. You can do this in any position, but you'll probably find it most comfortable to do while sitting in a chair or lying on your back. Squeeze your PC, hold for three seconds, then release. Repeat until you can build up to 100 at a time.
- According to Dr Cynthia Mervis Watson, co-author of *Love Potions: A Doctor's Guide to Aphrodisia*, the exercise should be done with your legs slightly apart rather than with your thighs clamped together. You will find that you are drawing your pelvis upwards, but if you find

the exercise tiring, it may be that you're also tensing your buttocks and abdomen; try to isolate only your PC muscles (see next step).
- Place a hand on your abdomen while contracting to ensure that it's relaxed. Inserting a finger into your vagina or placing a hand at the opening also helps identify the movement and confirm that you're squeezing the right muscles.

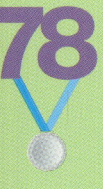

78
Now use your **pumped-up muscles** to milk him to orgasm. During sex, move your hips very slowly up and down his penis' shaft while squeezing your PCs so you can apply varying amounts of pressure to his organ. Mix in the pelvic moves worked on in tip 47 to get his penis to give you a massage at the same time.

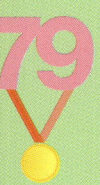

79
Crush him. When you're a groan away from climax, let loose by rapidly fluttering your PC muscles – squeezing faster with shorter pauses in between. Flex them five times quickly. The harder and more rapidly you squeeze, the stronger your and his orgasm will be.

30 Boogie slow and easy. Powerfully squeeze your PCs in a constricting manner to push him out. Repeat on the in-stroke, this time squeezing to pull him back in. Push out, constrict, pull in a little and push out and constrict again. When you've developed enough strength, you should be able to **keep it up all night** (get in top shape for this move with tip 45).

31 Twist to the corkscrew: With your knees bent, lie on top of your partner, who is on his back with his penis inside you. Resting on his chest, squeeze his penis and slowly circle your hips five times. Stop and release the squeeze. Then squeeze hard again and rotate your hips in the other direction. Continue this cycle until you are both ready to pop.

32 Get him to prod your hot spots. During sex, push down with your PCs to bring the front wall of your vagina down to meet his penis. This helps him **tickle your G-spot**. (Combine this with tip 46 to make this a Gold.)

33 Push it. Just add a gentle bearing-down motion to your Kegel contractions during sex, as if you were having a bowel movement. It sounds as sexy as a mental image of Robbie Coltrane naked, but it works.

LET'S GET PHYSICAL

Research has found that the couple who sweat together also sizzle together – they have sex more often and more orgasms when they do it. For an added incentive, do the sexercises naked.

84

Push-ups tone the chest and arms, making it a cinch to get on top (not to mention fuelling chandelier-swinging abilities). Kneel and place your palms in his hands. Slowly lower and push back up (kisses on the down move make a good incentive). Repeat ten times.

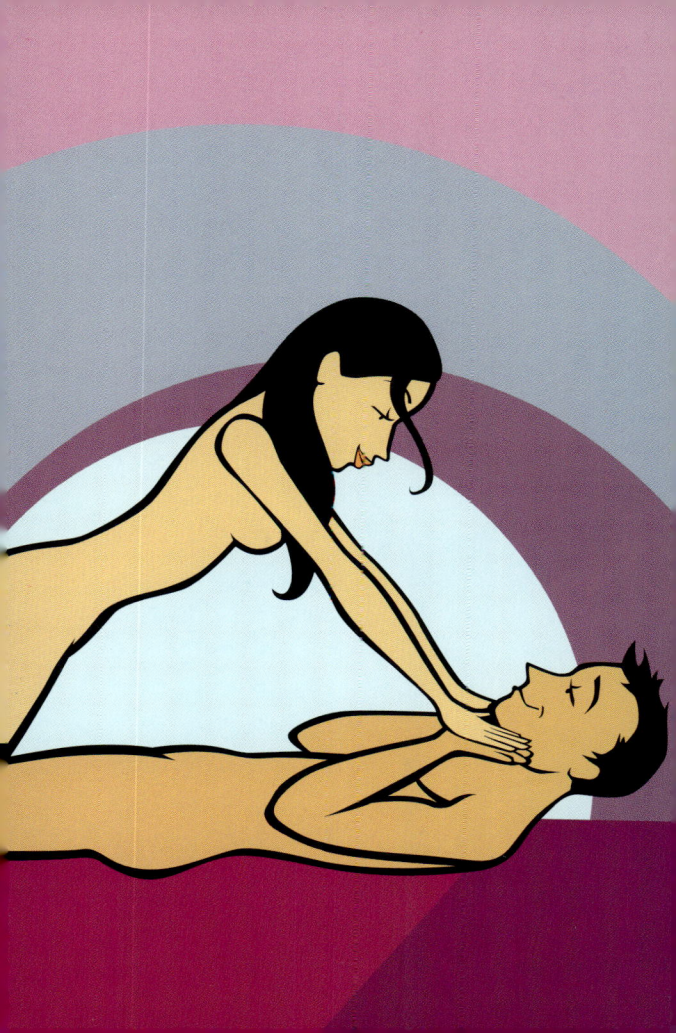

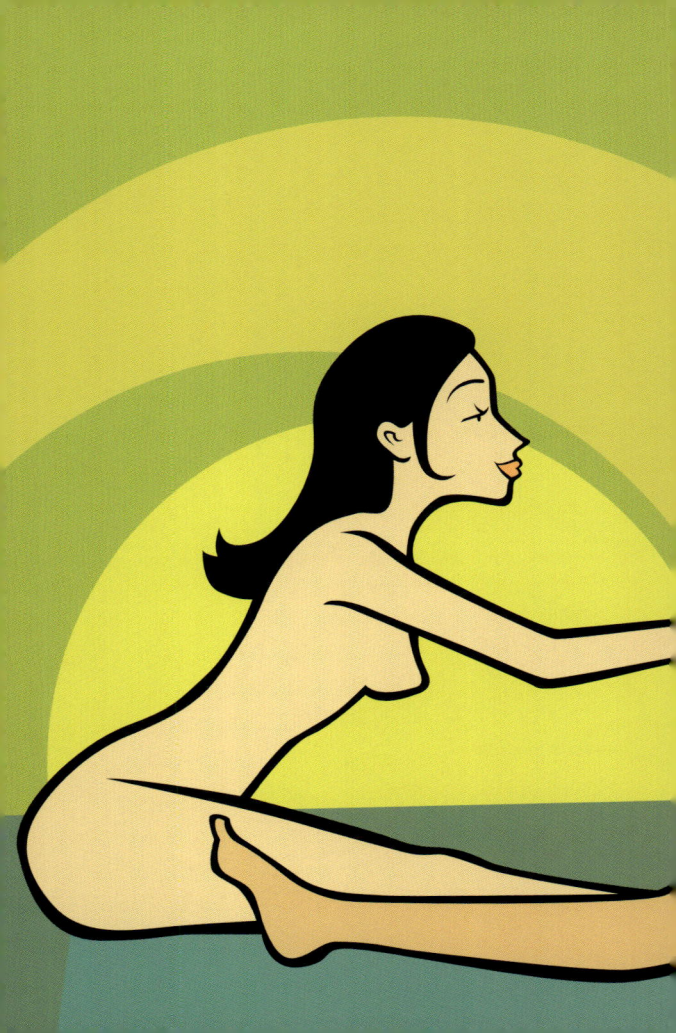

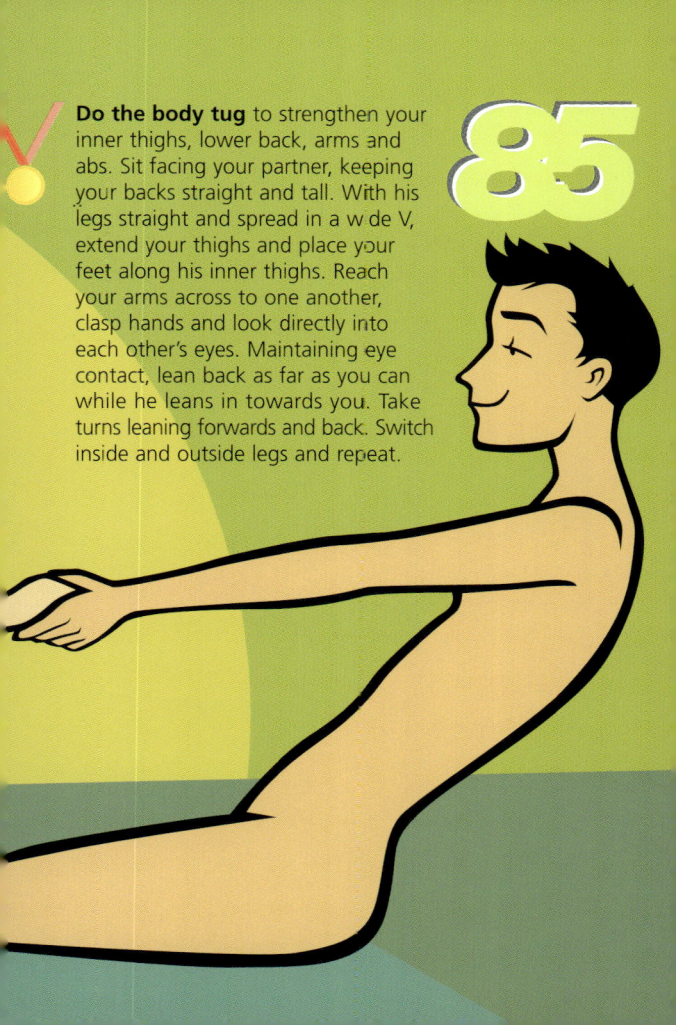

Do the body tug to strengthen your inner thighs, lower back, arms and abs. Sit facing your partner, keeping your backs straight and tall. With his legs straight and spread in a wide V, extend your thighs and place your feet along his inner thighs. Reach your arms across to one another, clasp hands and look directly into each other's eyes. Maintaining eye contact, lean back as far as you can while he leans in towards you. Take turns leaning forwards and back. Switch inside and outside legs and repeat.

85

Do a high-five for a whole-body workout. Stand very close to your partner, face to face. Both of you bend down into a squat, then jump up as high as you can and slap hands (and any other body parts you care to connect) together.

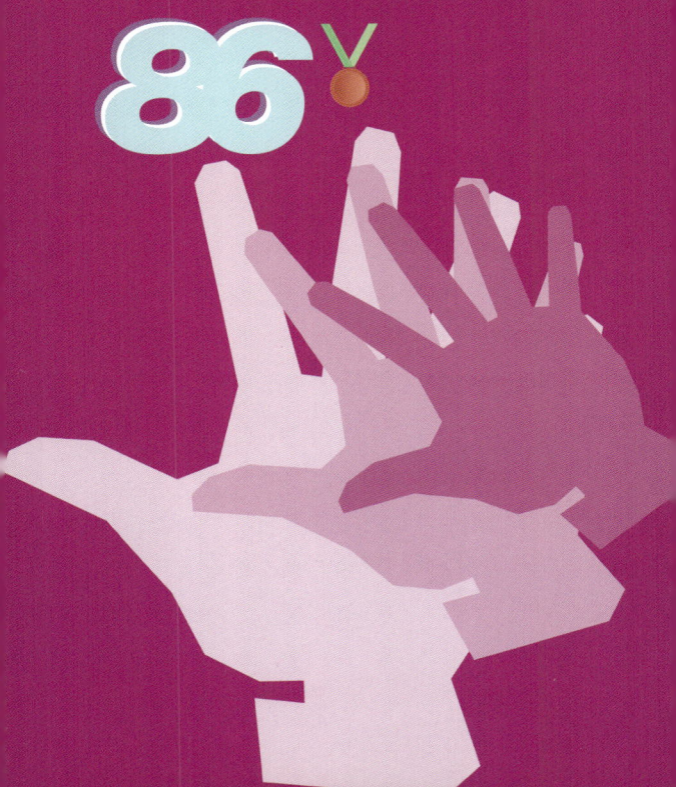

86

Do a better crunch. Instead of tip 50 (the abs workout), place your feet high on his chest (to prevent your back from arching) and contract your stomach, bringing your shoulders closer to your knees. Do two sets of 25 repetitions each.

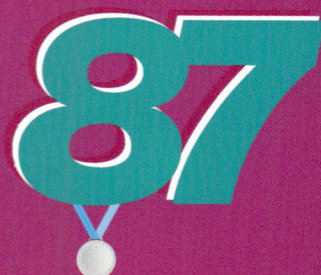

87

The pelvic tilt will keep hips, abs and thighs granite hard. Combine this with tip 77 and you'll be a sex engine. Lie on your back with your knees bent and your feet flat on the floor. Rest your arms by your sides and have your partner kneel beside you. As you raise your pelvis slowly off the floor, have him place his hands under you to help you hold the posture, making sure your hips and thighs are in line. Lower your pelvis to the floor and repeat.

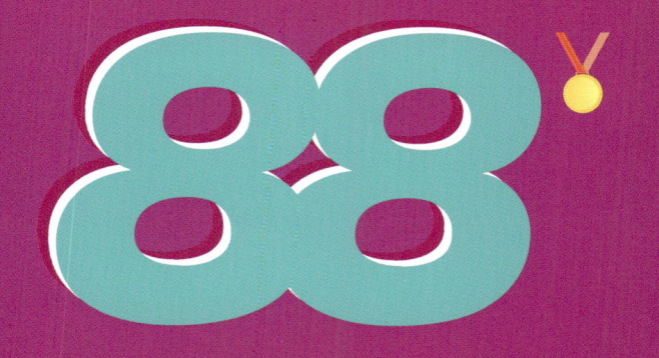

88

89

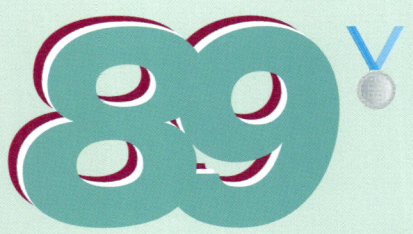

To **strengthen the lower back**, hang your upper body off the bed while he sits on your thighs to stabilize you. Then raise your torso just past horizontal, hold for one beat and lower. Repeat eight times.

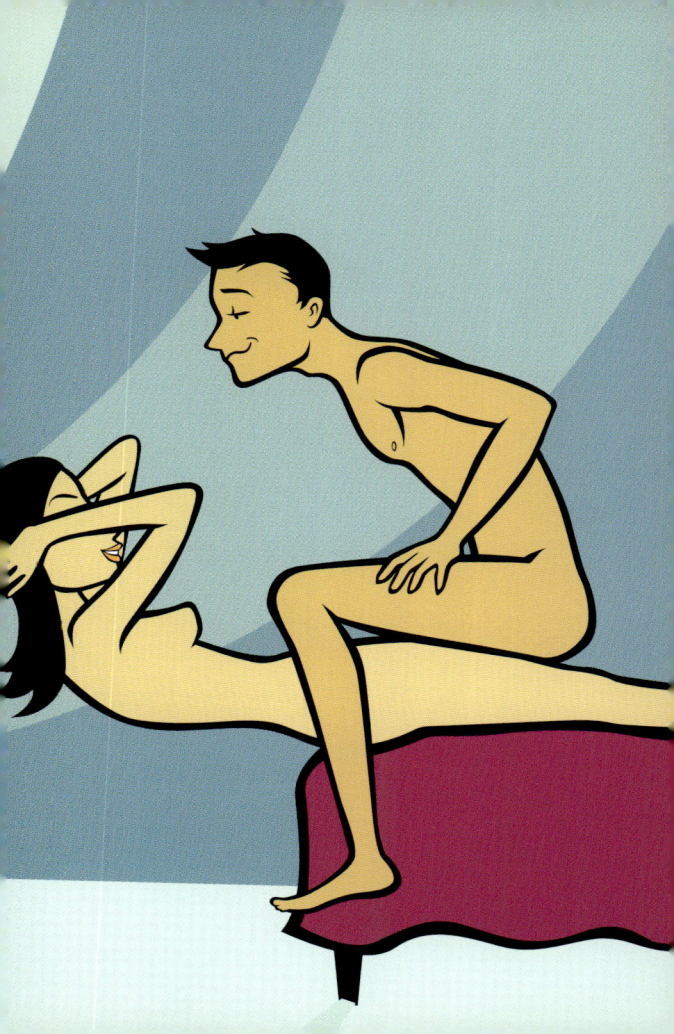

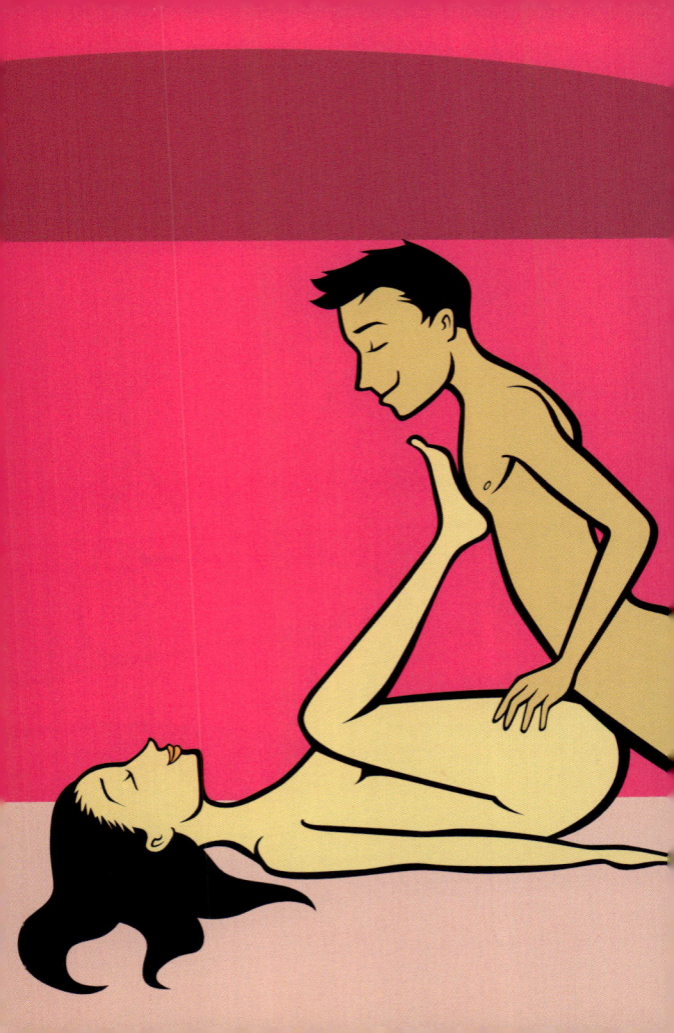

90

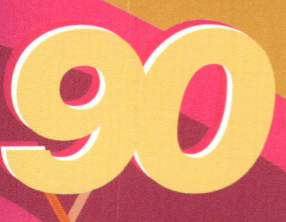

Place your feet high on his chest, supporting his body weight. Slowly lower him, bringing your knees to your chest. Push him back to the starting position (penetration is optional). Repeat five times.

Let him be your stretching rack. **Sit with your legs apart**, his feet above your ankles. As you relax forward, he gently pulls your arms to deepen the stretch (repeat twice).

91

PASSION POLE VAULTS

These moves count not only as great sex, but also great exercise. Get ready to do victory laps.

92 Press down*
TARGETS: shoulders
DO IT: Have your partner lie face up underneath you. He penetrates, then moves up and down by doing push-ups that are about half the range of movement of standard ones.

Push back 93
TARGETS: triceps
DO IT: Start from a sitting position on the floor. Lean back, supporting your weight with your hands behind you and your fingers pointing forward. Have your partner slip between your thighs with his knees and hands on the floor, his head just over your shoulder. Pick your bum off the ground. Once he lowers himself onto (and into) you, you do the work. From a bent-elbow starting position, thrust towards him by straightening your arms. Bend again. For more sextension, he can lean against you until you're supporting most of his weight.

94 Love curl*
TARGETS: Biceps
DO IT: Stand about 90 cm (3 ft) away from the wall, with your back to it. Lean your lower back and shoulders against the wall. He should lie on you with his chest to yours, his legs pressed against you and his penis inside you. Scoop your arms around him so your hands are resting against his shoulder blades. He leans back until your arms are extended (take care he doesn't slip out). Slowly curl him back to you. To make it easier, he can put his arms around you and help pull himself up.

Squatter* 95
TARGETS: Quads and hamstrings
DO IT: Have him squat low, leaning back against a wall. Squat over him, making sure you keep your knees bent at a right angle. Move up and down on his penis by pressing with your thighs (if this is too hard, you can give him some of your weight by putting your hands on his thighs).

* For these exercises you can easily switch places so he gets the workout as well.

96 Body bend

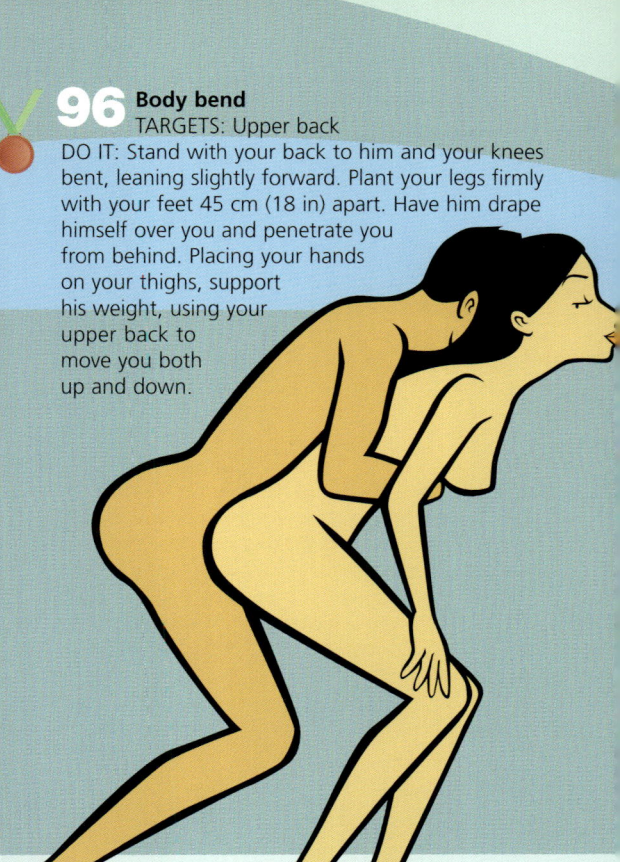

TARGETS: Upper back

DO IT: Stand with your back to him and your knees bent, leaning slightly forward. Plant your legs firmly with your feet 45 cm (18 in) apart. Have him drape himself over you and penetrate you from behind. Placing your hands on your thighs, support his weight, using your upper back to move you both up and down.

WORK IT

Slip these drills into your regular sex routine and he'll be bending over backwards to please you.

Break orgasm time records. During oral sex or intercourse, have your man support you by slipping his hands under your hips and lifting your pelvis up while you clench your bum muscles.

Put pressure on your abs. Your lower abdomen, just above the pubic hairline, is basically the outside of the inner clitoris. Squeezing the ab muscles intensifies the feeling inside. Do a mini sit-up during sex to tip you over the edge, as it will sandwich your inner clitoris between two hard surfaces (i.e., your tensed muscles and his penis). Note: make sure his penis or finger or whatever hard surface you're using is inserted first.

Open and close your legs during sex in small pumps. Doing this will trigger orgasm in two ways: first, closing your legs makes it easier to clench those thigh muscles (see tips 85, 88, 89 and 96 for strengthening exercises) which actually continue far enough to stimulate your inner clitoris. Second, opening and closing creates friction on the outer visible part of the clitoris and the inner folds of the vulva, which are rich in nerve bundles.

Section Five

WEEK FIVE: AN ORGASM A DAY

Newsflash: There is a pain-free way to boost looks, improve health, lower stress, make periods pain-free, reduce stress, lift moods, increase confidence and keep you in peak condition.

What is this unknown road to fabulousness?

Sex. And lots of it.

Okay, so you may not wake up with perfectly highlighted tresses, Brad Pitt and a fantastic TV sitcom contract. But it turns out that orgasms don't just feel good. They're also good for you. Because sexual arousal and orgasm involve the interplay of several body systems, it's now known that even a common-or-garden-variety shag does more for your physical wellbeing than a month-long holiday in Tahiti.

These are all the glorious reasons why getting physical will make you look and feel more beautiful (as if you needed an excuse to have more sex!).

THE LOOK OF LOVE

Making love is a painless way to make you look better (and much cheaper than visiting a spa!).

100
Who needs collagen when you have regular sex? A single make-out session can act as a luscious lip-puffer-upper that would make even Angelina Jolie bite her lips.

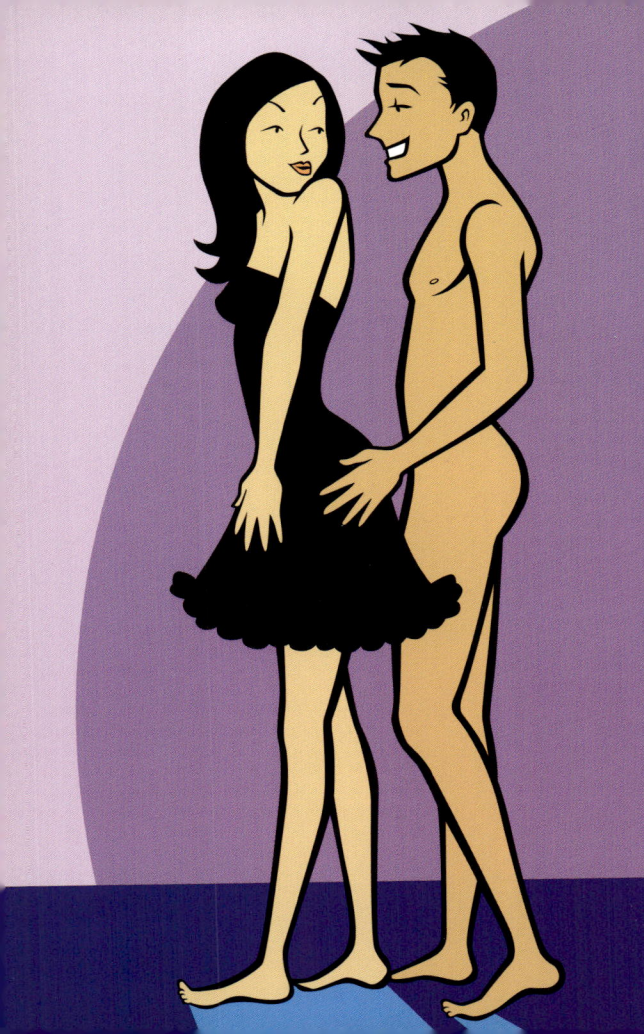

101

A snog a day keeps the cosmetic surgeon away. Kissing has been recognized as one of the best facial exercises around. Experts say that all that puckering tones up facial muscles, keeping you looking young and beautiful.

102

The only cover-up you need for your skin is **a sexy little number**. When Mr Desirable touches you, you get such an explosive rush that it sends blood rushing to the surface, making your heart beat faster and blood pressure rise. It's this rollercoaster of love that makes you positively glow after sex.

103

Toss away those AHA creams. According to an Ohio University study, orgasm increases your lymphocyte numbers (the cells responsible for fighting physical degeneration) – so regular climaxes could make you remain gorgeous well into old age – necessary when you consider tip 108!

Here's an inexpensive conditioner – sex is known to stimulate the hormones which give your hair a **healthy, shiny sheen**.

A little bit of sex can help you get away with shaving a few years off your age. A Royal Edinburgh Hospital in Scotland study found that sex helps you look between four and seven years younger because it helps you feel more content, sleep better and feel less stressed.

104 105 106

Regular lovemaking increases a woman's oestrogen level, which keeps the skin and vaginal tissues **supple, moist and glowing**.

GOOD MEDICINE

Love is the ultimate drug for staying healthy.

A bounce on the sheet will keep you committed to **your diet**: making love ups PEA levels (see tip 11), suppressing your appetite so much you can't even face a Cream Egg. And because you're getting oral gratification from kissing and nibbling parts of your lad's anatomy, your craving for food simply disappears.

107 108

The French call the orgasm **la petite mort** – the little death. But a little death now and then can help postpone the big death that's looming later on. A new study suggests that people who have sex twice a week live longer because sex helps raise the substances that lengthen life span – DHEA (see tip 111), oxytocin, endorphins (see tip 113) and growth hormone – and lower those that can shorten it – like cortisol and adrenaline.

Sex is like oxygen. Doing it kicks the respiratory system into overdrive. When you breathe deep and fast, your blood is enriched with oxygen, which nourishes all your organs and tissues.

Any kind of physical activity is going to **increase testosterone**. Sex is no exception. The magic male nectar has many happy effects. It makes both men and women's sex drive robust and fortifies bone and muscles. Some physicians believe that testosterone may even reduce joint inflammation and keep hearts healthy and good cholesterol high.

Sex delivers DHEA (dehydroepiandrosterone). The hormone spikes to levels three to five times higher than usual just before orgasm. This can perk up cognition, the immune system and bone growth, and inhibit tumour growth and fight depression.

A guy needs a **hosed-out prostrate gland** to function at peak level. Orgasm causes the muscles around the area to contract over and over, squeezing out excess fluids.

So much for the **'Not tonight, dear, I have a headache'** excuse. Doctors now credit orgasm as the ultimate analgesic, elevating the pain threshold and releasing endorphins (substances in the brain that are natural painkillers). This means sex can help relieve arthritic pain, whiplash pain and headache pain. It is also thought that orgasmic vaginal and pelvic contractions help relieve PMS cramps.

Doctors say a roll in the hay may keep sniffles away. In a recent under-the-covers investigation at Wilkes University in Pennsylvania, researchers found that students who **did the deed once a week** had about one-third higher levels of the antibody immunoglobulin A (the first line of defence against most diseases – colds, flu, even cancer) than their more celibate peers.

If you're lucky enough to have **sex three times a week** – nothing fancy, just a modest merger – you'll burn about 7,500 calories every year. That's the equivalent of jogging 75 miles. And remember – these are calories spent before you even hit the play button on your Buns of Steel workout video.

1617

During arousal and orgasm there is what's called **myotonia** (contraction by any other name) **of the muscles**. So, the more lifting, spinning and thrusting, the better from a muscle-building point of view.

You'll also get toned when you do these moves (who needs aerobics?):

The Move: Body Buffer

Oral sex (you): jaw, neck, thighs
69: abs, bum, neck, jaw
Missionary: thighs, bum
Spoons: bottom, abs
Rear entry: abs, back, bum, thighs, hamstrings
You on top: bum, thighs, abs

ATTITUDE ADJUSTER

The special effects sex has on your brain are just as important as the physical rewards. Here are the major mental extras:

Sex is like a natural Prozac. Because arousal and orgasm shoot pleasure-inducing endorphin bullets into the brain (see tip 113), they are believed to alter the chemistry thought to cause depression, according to a study by New Mexico Highlands University.

Have an orgasm and **learn to love yourself**. A study of 164 female and male exercisers at Connecticut College in New London found that those who had sex regularly had significantly more self-esteem than non-nookie players.

There's plenty of research to show that stress is one of the most common causes of **sexual dysfunction** and lack of drive. But there's MORE research to indicate that sex can be a very effective way of reducing stress. It chills you out, suffuses you with a profound feeling of wellbeing and relaxation, and reduces the internal chatter.

Being sexual **keeps the brain curious and functioning creatively**, according to a study by the Royal Edinburgh Hospital in Scotland. Enjoy …